ASTHMA

Megan Gressor was a health reporter for *Family Circle* magazine for several years and has worked in senior editorial positions for other leading publications, including *Reader's Digest, Woman's Day* and *Better Homes & Gardens*. She is the author of several popular health books.

ASTHMA
Breathe Easy

MEGAN GRESSOR

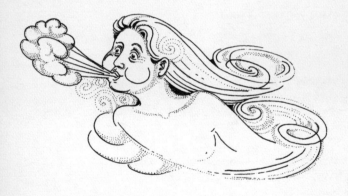

ROBINSON
London

Robinson Publishing Ltd
7 Kensington Church Court
London W8 4SP

First published in Great Britain by
Robinson Publishing Ltd 1995

Published in Australia by
Gore & Osment Publications Pty Ltd

Copyright © Megan Gressor 1992
Copyright © Gore & Osment Publications Pty Ltd

ISBN 1–85487–386–5

A copy of the British Library Cataloguing in Publication
Data is available from the British Library

Note
This book is not a substitute for your doctor's or health
professional's advice, and the publishers and author
cannot accept liability for any injury or loss to any
person acting or refraining from action as a result of
the material in this book. Before commencing any
health treatment, always consult your own doctor.

Printed and bound in the EC

Contents

Introduction

Asthma is on the increase in Britain. Around one in every 10 adults suffers from asthma and the rate for children is even more alarming, with one in 7 of them suffering from the disease at some stage of their childhood.

Our asthma rates aren't just bad, they're getting worse. Respiratory experts warn that they are not only seeing more cases of asthma, but that those cases they see have increased in severity over the past 10 years or so. The majority of asthmatics have fairly mild asthma, being more inconvenienced than seriously impaired by their symptoms. But asthma can be a killer.

Many people, including asthmatics themselves, fail to realise just how serious a disease it can be. Part of the problem is that many asthmatics look and feel fine most of the time – until an attack strikes, seemingly out of the blue. Even after an attack is triggered, asthmatics may fail to realise its potential seriousness and to seek appropriate medical attention. Delay in seeking hospital treatment is said to be a factor in as many as 30 per cent of asthma deaths. Relatively few of these deaths occur in children, however, despite their high prevalence of asthma. This could be because we tend to take our children's health far more seriously than we do our own.

There is no 'cure' for asthma, though it can be effectively treated. But, for treatment to be successful, it is vital that adult asthmatics pay attention to their condition, which means listening to what their lungs are trying to tell them. Far too many asthmatics:

- Rely on bronchodilators (medication, such as Ventolin, Salbutamol and Bricanyl, that relieves asthma symptoms but doesn't treat the underlying problem).
- Neglect other, *preventative* medication.
- Fail to monitor their lung capacity.
- Do not avoid factors which aggravate their asthma.

They may pay a high penalty for such self-neglect. If their asthma is not treated and controlled, they could suffer permanent lung damage, and even death.

As medical supervision is very important, this book should not be seen as a substitute for a doctor's advice and care. Rather, its aim is to help asthmatics and their families to understand their condition, and through that understanding, learn how to control it – rather than be controlled by it. Armed by this knowledge, they, and those around them, should be able to breathe easy.

Chapter 1
What Is Asthma?

Asthma is a disease characterised by the narrowing of the airways of the lungs. With this disease, three things happen, all of which contribute to this narrowing: the **muscles** of these airways tighten and go into spasm; the **lining** of the airways swells up; and excessive **mucus** is produced.

All of these make breathing difficult, which is why breathlessness is a key sign of asthma. The characteristic asthmatic wheeze is the sound made by air being exhaled through the narrowed airways – in a manner similar to the way that air forced through the narrow neck of a deflating balloon makes a loud, whining noise.

WHAT CAUSES ASTHMA?

Why the airways go into spasm in this way is not really understood. It is usually in response to an **irritant** – such as cigarette smoke, fly spray or cold air – or a **sensitiser** – such as infection, certain chemicals or **allergens** (substances which trigger allergic reactions). The majority of people cope with these without undue problems, apart from some temporary coughing or spluttering. But the airways of asthmatics seem to have become hypersensitive ('twitchy'), and overreact to irritants and sensitisers. The term asthma refers to this hypersensitive tendency, not to acute attacks as such, and people who have it are called asthmatics. That tendency still remains even after attacks may have ceased, as they often do after childhood. This is why some people may have attacks after many years free of them.

WHAT TRIGGERS ATTACKS?

While we may not know what causes asthmatics' airways to become hypersensitive in this fashion, we do know that certain factors can trigger asthma attacks. Such trigger factors can include the following:

- Chest and throat infections and colds.
- Exercise, especially running.
- Cold weather and temperature changes.
- Exposure to strong smells and cigarette smoke.
- Excitement, stress and emotional upset.
- Allergic reactions: to dust, pollen, animal hair, etc.
- Exposure to certain substances encountered at the workplace.

Symptoms of an Asthma Attack

A full-blown asthma attack can be a terrifying experience, and victims may feel as though they are suffocating. They inhale in short gasps and exhale in long, noisy wheezes, as they battle to get breath through the blocked airways.

Their lower ribs may contract sharply as they inhale (this is particularly noticeable in young children), their pulse races and, during severe attacks, their lips and other parts may turn blue from lack of oxygen.

Other less dramatic symptoms they may experience include:

- Tightness of the chest.
- A dry cough.
- Anxiety and shakiness.

Symptoms are often worst on waking or during the night.

FACT FILE

Seasonal Wheeze?
Many people believe that asthma is more prevalent in **spring**, during the pollen season (pollen being an asthma trigger). But in cities, attacks are more likely to peak during **winter**, particularly in children, due to colds and infections.

WHO IS AT RISK?

Asthma can strike at any age, at any time. It can first occur in babyhood and is common in young children; but can also develop quite late in life (this is called **late onset asthma**).

Boys are at greater risk of childhood asthma, while women seem more susceptible to the adult variety.

There is a hereditary factor – the tendency to hypersensitivity is genetically determined – which is why the doctor diagnosing your asthma may ask if it runs in your family. Asthma is linked with certain other allergic-type conditions, such as eczema, hay fever and urticaria (inflammation of the skin). These also have a hereditary basis. So if your great-uncle Fred had hay fever and your mother has eczema, you could be a candidate for asthma.

FACT FILE

Did You Know?
Asthma is on the increase. According to the National Health Survey carried out by the Australian Bureau of Statistics, the proportion of the population experiencing asthma as a long-term condition quadrupled between 1978 and 1990. Nearly half a million working days are lost to asthma, together with other respiratory complaints, a year.

THE ASTHMA/ALLERGY CONNECTION

Asthma itself can be an allergic reaction to specific substances, as we've seen. This is called **extrinsic** asthma, and is more commonly encountered in children. Asthma which starts late in life is less likely to have an allergic basis.

WHAT HAPPENS DURING AN ALLERGIC REACTION?

When the body encounters an allergen – by inhaling, eating or touching it – it reacts by activating **mast cells**. These are special cells found throughout the body which are in effect tiny chemical factories, manufacturing substances involved in the body's **immune response** (destruction of infections and 'foreign' objects). One of these chemicals is **histamine**, which reacts to allergens by stimulating mucus production and tightening the muscles of the airways – which can trigger an asthma attack.

Anti-histamines, medications which block the action of histamine, are effective against some allergic conditions, such as hay fever, but not against asthma.

ALLERGY TESTING

Because of this allergic aspect, the doctor diagnosing your asthma may decide to order allergy tests – either a **skin test** or **RAST test**. With skin testing, a small quantity of suspect substances – which could be such common allergens as dust mites, pollen or animal dander (hair, skin scales, fur and feathers) – is smeared on the skin, which is then pierced. If the skin reacts by itching, reddening and/or swelling, you seem to be allergic to the substance in question (seem, because skin testing is not necessarily always reliable). The RAST (short for radioallergosorbent) test is a blood test which detects the presence of allergic antibodies in the blood.

Some people know exactly what they're allergic to, because their reaction to it is so immediate and intense. Others may not be so sure, particularly if they're allergic to a number of substances, or the allergic reaction takes longer to develop after exposure. If you can identify the offending item(s), you're more able to avoid exposure to it (or them), and thereby miss out on unpleasant reactions. (See next two chapters.)

HOW YOUR LUNGS WORK

To understand fully what is happening during an asthma attack, you have to know how your respiratory system – 'breathing apparatus' – really works, and what can go wrong.

Every minute of our lives we inhale 6 litres plus of air required to supply the body's cells with the oxygen they need to function. Breathing seems a simple enough business – we do it thousands of times a day, after all, even when we're asleep – but if we stopped for even a few minutes, our tissues, starved of the life-giving oxygen, would start to die.

With each breath we take, air is drawn in through the nose, which warms, filters and moistens it – in effect, conditioning it – before it passes down to the **pharynx** (the gateway to both the stomach and the lungs, which connects the back of the throat with the oesophagus). From there, the air moves down to the **larynx** (Adam's apple or voice box), and then into the **trachea** (windpipe), a cartilage-ringed tube which runs down into the chest and divides into the right and left main **bronchus** (plural bronchi).

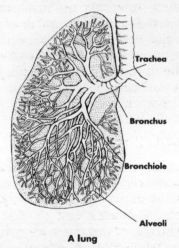

A lung

These **bronchi** lead into each lung, where they branch off into a network of smaller and smaller airways. These are often represented as a sort of inverted tree, with the trunk-like bronchi dividing into the smaller **bronchioles**, which in turn branch into clusters of tiny **alveoli**. These are the lungs' air sacs, where the **exchange of gases** takes place. This is the vital function that is the purpose of breathing: oxygen from the air passes through the alveoli's thin membranes into the blood; and carbon dioxide from the blood passes back through those membranes and up the airways, to be exhaled when we breathe out. This feat requires the involvement of more than 300,000,000 alveoli, with a total estimated surface area equivalent to that of a tennis court!

This whole marvellous structure is self-cleansing. Foreign bodies, such as dust and other irritants, are trapped by **mucus**, a sticky substance secreted by the **mucosa**, a layer of special cells lining the inner walls of the respiratory system. The trapped impurities are swept away from the lungs by tiny hair-like filaments called **cilia**. The cilia move in a continuous wave-like motion, brushing the mucus-encased foreign bodies back up towards the mouth, where they are swallowed. Most of us are unaware of how much mucus this process produces. We just swallow, automatically, dozens of times a day.

The production of mucus is essential to keep the airways clean. More mucus is produced when they are exposed to irritating substances, such as cigarette smoke. Coughing – a normal response to such irritants – helps to clear that extra mucus. Asthmatics' hypersensitive airways over-react to irritants by producing too much mucus, further blocking airways

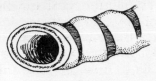

Normal airway

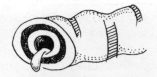

**During an asthma attack.
The muscles of the airways tighten,
their linings swell, and excess mucus
is produced.**

already narrowed by muscle spasm. That is why coughing – to try to get rid of all that mucus – is such a key symptom of asthma. It is sometimes the only symptom.

Two body chemicals are involved in the contraction of the bronchi experienced during an asthma attack. They are:

- **Histamine:** Released from the body's mast cells after exposure to allergens.
- **Acetyl choline:** This is released from the vagus nerve which controls the bronchial muscle.

Both these substances contract the bronchial muscle. Other substances naturally present in the body relax it – such as **adrenalin**, manufactured by the adrenal glands, which plays a crucial part in the body's fight or flight reaction to stress. Adrenalin opens up the airways, allowing a greater oxygen intake to aid escape from a dangerous situation. Some asthma medications work by mimicking the action of adrenalin. More about medication in Chapter 5.

Chapter 2
Asthma Triggers

'Everything gives you cancer – there's no cure, there's no answer,' sings Joe Jackson in his ironic hit song *Cancer*. Just replace the word cancer with asthma and you'll have the asthmatics' national anthem, for it can sometimes seem that almost <u>anything</u> can trigger an attack – and nobody quite knows why. One individual's asthma may be triggered by a substance or event that leaves others quite unaffected.

However, if you can identify the factor(s) triggering your asthma, you're halfway towards heading off an attack. Once you recognise the culprit, you can reduce the risks by avoiding exposure to it as much as possible.

Let's look at some common trigger factors in more detail.

DUST MITES

These nasty little creatures lurk in dust deposits and eat human skin scales, which we shed continuously. They thrive in warm, humid conditions and are particularly prevalent in bedrooms. They are to be found in bedding (particularly feather pillows and down-filled duvets), mattresses, curtains, upholstered furniture and carpets. You're unlikely ever to see one unless you own a microscope, for they are minuscule – an estimated 42,000 of them can be found in a single ounce of mattress dust. Inhaling their droppings irritates the airways, which is why medical authorities may recommend a mite eradication campaign for some asthmatics. Not everybody will find their asthma improved by the following measures, so you should seek your doctor's advice before embarking on such a campaign. Its effectiveness can't be guaranteed even so; however, it can certainly do no harm – and will at least leave your home sparkling clean and dust-free!

A Dust Mite

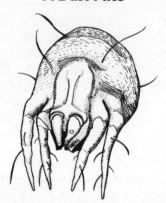

A mere 25 grams of mattress dust may hold up to 42,000 of these microscopic creatures

- Keep dust mite numbers down by vacuuming frequently, particularly around and under the bed (remember that any sort of cleaning that raises dust can trigger asthma attacks, so cover your face when vacuuming and sweeping; and use a filter on the vacuum cleaner).
- Wherever possible, choose bare floors (lino, wood, tiles) rather than wall-to-wall carpet, which provides an ideal environment for dust and mould.
- Plastic-covered foam mattresses harbour less dust than the cloth-covered padded variety. The latter can be covered in zippered plastic covers. Some asthmatics swear by waterbeds, which, of course, harbour no dust at all.
- Choose holland blinds rather than dust-catching venetians.
- Avoid fluffy woollen blankets and down-filled quilts and pillows. Cotton or synthetic bedclothes are better. Launder bedclothes and curtain material frequently.
- Vinyl furniture harbours less dust than fabric-upholstered chairs and sofas.

POLLEN

Pollen – that fine golden powder that flowers produce to fertilise one another – is a powerful allergen. Carried on the wind, it makes many (non-asthmatic) people's noses run and eyes stream, and it can cause serious problems for asthmatics. There's not much you can do to minimise your exposure to pollen, so it's just as well that the pollen season is brief, just a few weeks in springtime. During that time, you should try to:

- Stay indoors as much as possible, and keep windows closed.
- Keep away from grassy areas.
- Never volunteer to mow the lawn!

MOULD

Like pollen, mould can trigger asthma attacks if inhaled. Mould is the grey-green fungus to be found on decomposing food and vegetable matter, plants, walls, bathroom and laundry fittings, poorly aired clothing and textiles. It is common in damp and poorly ventilated areas. Before embarking on a mould-reduction campaign, you should first discuss with your doctor whether mould is in fact the culprit triggering *your* asthma. If so, here's how to minimise your exposure:

- Keep the house as dry and well-ventilated as possible.
- Use bleach and mould-killer to eliminate mould on tiles and grouting, on shower curtains and inside cupboards, and around sinks, basins and toilets.
- Choose lino, tiles or wooden floors. Carpets can be breeding grounds for mould as well as dust.

- Regularly check your air-conditioner filter for mould.
- Don't let rotting leaves accumulate outdoors, and keep away from compost heaps.

INFECTIONS

Viral infections (colds, flu, bronchitis and so on) can trigger asthma attacks because they irritate the airways and cause them to contract, as well as provoke mucus production – all of which is bad news for already hypersensitive airways. Children are particularly susceptible to viral infections because of their relatively undeveloped immune systems. Their asthma may worsen in autumn and winter, when such infections are more common. Viral infections do not respond to antibiotics. There's not a lot you can do to avoid them – other than giving a wide berth to obviously infected individuals and building up your resistance by looking after yourself (eating good food, getting enough rest and regular exercise and avoiding stress).

SMOKING

Cigarette smoke irritates the airways and damages the lungs. Stopping smoking is the biggest single favour asthmatics can do for themselves. Family members should refrain from smoking, too, because passive smoking can also trigger attacks. It's thought that the present epidemic of childhood asthma may be caused, in part, by exposure to parents' cigarette smoke: the incidence of asthma is at least 50 per cent higher in children whose parents both smoke than in children of non-smokers. There is evidence that pregnant women who smoke have babies with a greater susceptibility to asthma. Passive smoking is not confined to the home, of course. At work, try to avoid colleagues' smoke as much as possible (easier in these days of smoke-free offices). Ask them to refrain from smoking around you, or request a move so that you can be seated next to non-smokers. Don't be afraid to be assertive; you should not have to tolerate having workmates' smoke blown in your face (and into your lungs).

ENVIRONMENTAL POLLUTION

Belching smoke stacks, car exhaust, the sulphur dioxide emitted in diesel fumes – these are all fixtures of modern industrialised living. Each of them takes a toll on your lungs (as can that more old-fashioned form of environmental pollution, the humble open fireplace). Industrial pollution may be partly to blame for the increased prevalence of asthma, though the jury is still out on this one. If it is to blame, there isn't much you can do about it, apart from moving house to an area of lower pollution – expensive and possibly ineffective, as there's no guarantee that the asthma will clear up else-where.

OCCUPATIONAL HAZARDS

Some people suffer from what is described as occupational asthma. This means that certain chemicals and substances they encounter on the job are triggering their asthma, which follows a typical pattern: they feel worse during the week and recover on weekends, when they are away from work. Such substances can include:

- Isocynates (used to make polyurethanes, plastics and paints).
- Formaldehyde.
- Acid anhydrides, used in the plastic industry.
- Vapours from soldering fluxes (colophony).
- Certain reactive dyes used to dye cotton and synthetic fibres, and in hair colourings.
- Platinum salts (used in electroplating, photography, the manufacture of jewellery and fluorescent screens).
- Diazonium salts (used in photocopiers).
- Wood dust.
- Grain dust. (This can make a baker's life difficult – there is a type of occupational asthma called 'baker's asthma' – because of problems they experience from frequently inhaling flour.)

The solution to occupational asthma may seem simple: change your job! The logic of this seems particularly compelling when you realise that continuous exposure to an asthma trigger over time increases the airways' sensitivity and worsens the asthma. However, what seems logical is not always practicable, particularly in times of recession and high unemployment. Your job may be making you wheeze, but it's also paying the rent and putting food on the table.

When leaving the job is not an option, medication may be the solution to occupational asthma. Changes to the workplace can reduce your exposure. Better ventilation, improved cleanliness to control dust, and safer handling and disposal of irritating substances should all be considered. Your union or health-and-safety officer may be able to advise on modifications to the workplace and work practices to reduce your contact with irritants.

TEMPERATURE CHANGES

Sudden changes (particularly drops) in temperature can trigger asthma attacks. This is why children rushing about in the early evening, when the air cools rapidly, frequently suffer attacks. (Exercise can be another trigger – see p.19 – so the combination of wild play and cold air doubles the risks of an attack.)

Climatic variations – sudden fluctuations

between hot and cold – also provoke asthma attacks.

Once again, there's not much you can do about the weather – apart from migrating to an area where it's less changeable, which seems another rather drastic solution. However, a home heater or air-conditioner with a thermostat which allows you to maintain the air temperature indoors at a steady level could be a worthwhile investment, particularly in the bedroom. This will keep the room warm throughout the night, when the risks of attack are greatest. As a bonus, air-conditioners reduce relative humidity, which in turn should reduce the local dust mite population!

EXERCISE

We breathe more rapidly and heavily when we exercise, and this irritates and dries out hypersensitive airways. Any sort of exercise can trigger asthma attacks, though sustained exercise, such as running or football (as opposed to more stop/start sports like tennis), is more likely to provoke an attack. Children are particularly susceptible to exercise-induced asthma.

Exercise is one trigger factor that's not necessarily a good idea to avoid. This is because regular, moderate exercise is very important in maintaining general good health. Exercise-induced asthma may be prevented by taking medication before and during the exercise. More information about this in Chapter 8.

FACT FILE

Test Case:
In July, 1991, Allan Blackfield, a councillor on the City of Hawthorn Council, brought a case before the Victorian Equal Opportunity Tribunal in Australia, claiming that he had developed asthma after attending council conferences which featured 'excessively heavy' smoking. This was believed to be the first case of its kind in which a worker claimed to have been discriminated against because his employer didn't provide a smoke-free environment.

PETS

Animal dander – hair, skin scales, fur and feathers – can cause allergic reactions and asthma attacks. The risks are greater with cats than dogs. This is because cats lick themselves continuously, leading to a concentration of saliva on their fur. Some asthmatics are allergic to this saliva, and handling cats can trigger attacks. One solution to this problem (if you don't want to get rid of the cat) is to wash it regularly to avoid saliva build-up. While the first impulse of a family with a newly diagnosed asthmatic member might well be to get rid of all pets, animal dander is not a particularly strong asthma trigger (compared, say, with pollen or dust mites). You may want to give the pet a reprieve until you see exactly how much effect it has on the asthmatic. Try sending it away for a few weeks, and gauge the asthmatic's reaction on its return. If it's bad, you may have to trade it in for a goldfish. If you decide to keep the pet, ban such unwise habits as letting it sleep on your bed at night. Refrain from handling it, and keep it outside as much as possible.

MEDICATION

Aspirin can trigger asthma attacks, as can certain other medications, such as the beta-blockers prescribed to lower blood pressure. Look out for aspirin added to many over-the-counter cold, flu and indigestion preparations. Get into the habit of reading labels on medications; when in doubt, ask your doctor or pharmacist. Drug guides and compendiums, available in your library or from bookshops, list adverse reactions to prescription and over-the-counter drugs. It's not a bad idea to get into the habit of looking up any medication you're taking, to see if it's contra-indicated (not recommended) for asthmatics. As well, certain colourings used for some medications (particularly yellow, orange or green) can trigger attacks. More about problems with colourings and food additives in the next chapter.

STRESS

'Asthma is something that only happens to nervy people – it's all in the mind.' This is a common, annoying and dangerous myth about asthma. It is a physical disease, with all-too-concrete symptoms.

However, like many illnesses, it can be triggered or worsened by stress. Asthma attacks in children, for instance, have been linked to parental conflict, marriage break-ups and other traumatic life events. It's unrealistic to expect to go through life without experiencing any stress at all, and this is one trigger factor you're going to find hard to avoid.

However, while you can't prevent stressful events happening to you, you can learn to control your reaction to them.

Check out your own tension level: are your muscles often tight, causing pain and fatigue? Is your jaw habitually clenched, resulting in headache, jaw pain and toothache? When not using your hands, do you often unconsciously ball them into fists?

Other symptoms of stress include digestive upsets, insomnia, depression and sexual problems. If you've ticked one or more of these, it sounds as though you need to learn how to relax. It could be worth investigating stress-management courses, relaxation classes, yoga, meditation or any other form of therapy or activity that helps you to relax and unwind.

Not every asthmatic will find his or her asthma improved by relaxation therapy. However, learning to control your reaction to stress is recommended for many conditions, not just asthma, and can certainly do no harm. Many people find it makes them feel better, mentally as well as physically, so it's probably worth giving it a go.

Since stress can trigger asthma, staying as relaxed as possible between attacks may help to decrease their number and severity. Once an asthma attack has been triggered, you may find yourself in a vicious stress cycle; the panic caused by being unable to breathe properly increases your anxiety, which in turn exacerbates your symptoms. It follows that you should try to keep as calm as possible during an attack. This, of course, is easier said than done; being unable to breathe properly is one of the most alarming human experiences, and it's hard to keep your head when you can't draw breath. It may be easier if you have learned relaxation therapy and breathing exercises. For more, read on.

FACT FILE

Did You Know?
Asthma is rare among Eskimos. Though their environment is very cold, it is also relatively free of dust and the dust mites that thrive in warm, humid conditions.

HYPERVENTILATION

This is another common response to stress which is of particular significance to asthmatics. Hyperventilation is a bad breathing habit which involves taking fast, shallow breaths, using the muscles of the upper chest and neck.

This results in an excessive intake of oxygen and decreased levels of carbon dioxide in the blood. Hyperventilation can cause quite dramatic symptoms, including dizziness, tight chest, rapid heartbeat, light-headedness, breathlessness (sometimes called 'air hunger') and sighing. Some of these symptoms sound familiar, don't they? It's not surprising that people sometimes think they're having asthma attacks when, in fact, they are hyperventilating.

Everyone who hyperventilates is not an asthmatic, but asthmatics are particularly prone to it. This is because the narrowing of the small airways stimulates the brain's respiratory centre to respond with faster, deeper breathing. This can cause bronchospasm (sudden tightening of the muscles of the airways) and asthma attacks. You may well find that the stress and tension of everyday living is making you habitually hyperventilate without necessarily being aware of it, thus increasing your risk of attacks.

Breathing exercises – learning how to breathe from the diaphragm and abdomen, rather than shallow breathing using neck and upper chest muscles – could help to train you out of hyperventilating; ask your doctor or physiotherapist to teach you how to do them. Learning to control your breathing is a form of relaxation therapy in itself.

Chapter 3
Asthma and Diet

We live in an age of food fads, and you may encounter people or publications advocating particular (sometimes quite peculiar) diets to treat or 'cure' asthma. However, asthmatics should not see themselves as invalids, requiring special foods or odd eating plans. In general, they should follow the same healthy eating guidelines recommended for everyone. That is:

- More complex carbohydrates – vegetables, fruit, wholegrains and bread
- Moderate amounts of protein – fish, chicken, eggs, lean meat
- Reduced amounts of fat and sugar
- Less salt

This being said, however, there are certain substances, principally food additives, which asthmatics may be advised to *avoid* because of their tendency to trigger attacks.

FOOD ALLERGIES

Some foods, however healthy, can trigger allergic reactions. Such food allergies can trigger asthma attacks, though this is relatively rare. Suspect foods include egg whites, chocolate and peanuts, though sensitivity to specific substances can vary widely with the individual. The allergic reaction is likely to occur quite soon after eating (within 30 minutes or so) and is demonstrated in symptoms like:

- Wheezing and coughing
- Blocked or runny nose
- Swelling lips
- Vomiting, stomach pains
- Itching skin

Testing for Food Allergies

Simple observation may indicate which food is the culprit; if not, it may be identified by what is called a **challenge test**. This should be done under medical supervision, possibly in hospital. The individual abstains from suspect foods for a period of time, during which lung function is carefully monitored. The food is then eaten, and lung function is monitored for some hours afterwards. If it deteriorates, you've identified a food to avoid in future.

If you have no idea which food is provoking your reaction, your doctor may recommend an **elimination diet**. This involves going on to an extremely simple, limited diet (basically rice, fruit and vegetables) for a period of time, then gradually reintroducing different types of food, one after another. Again, your lung function will be monitored and your reaction to each food should identify those to which you are allergic.

FOOD ADDITIVES

It is more likely to be a food additive (preservative or colouring) which is causing the problem, however. Certain additives are known asthma triggers. These are Metabisulphite; Monosodium Glutamate (MSG); and Tartrazine.

Metabisulphite (Approved Additives Nos 211, 220, 221, 222, 223, 224)

This is a preservative added to various foods to maintain colour and inhibit the growth of bacteria.

It may be found in:

- Glass-bottled fruit juices
- Champagne
- Red wine
- White wine
- Beer/cider
- Vinegar
- Some dried fruits, such as apricots and apples (though *not* prunes, sultanas, currants or raisins)
- Fruit-flavoured yoghurt
- Dried vegetables, such as dried mashed potato

- Processed potato chips and crisps
- Pickles
- Sausages
- Cooked meats
- Lettuce

FACT FILE

Milk and Mucus

Many people believe that drinking cows' milk stimulates mucus production, and thus should be avoided by asthmatics. There is no particular evidence that this is the case, however.

On the subject of milk, breast-fed babies seem to suffer fewer allergies than those fed on other types of milk. Given the asthma-allergy connection, could this mean that bottle-fed babies are more at risk of developing asthma? Research has not yet provided an answer. But medical authorities recommend breast feeding when possible because of its many health benefits, including the mother's own antibodies boosting the baby's immune system.

Monosodium Glutamate (Approved Additive No 621)

This is a flavour-enhancer added to many processed foods. It is a well-known, even notorious, ingredient of many Asian dishes.

Soy sauce and hot, spicy sauces, those other standbys of Asian cookery, are high in MSG. Many other flavourings and seasonings also contain MSG, so should be looked upon with a generally suspicious eye.

Despite its well-publicised dangers, however, MSG is less likely to trigger an asthma attack than metabisulphite. And it can be difficult to work out whether MSG is to blame, given that attacks may occur some time (up to 12 hours later) after eating foods containing MSG.

Foods containing MSG may include:

- Prepared soups
- Potato crisps
- Savoury biscuits
- Frankfurts, pies and sausage rolls
- Cooked meats
- Commercial frozen meats
- Commercial gravy mixes
- Stock cubes
- Some commercial seasonings
- Sandwich spreads such as Vegemite and Marmite
- Canned meats, canned vegetables (in sauce)
- Tomato sauce and tomato paste

Related additives to avoid include: L-Glutamic acid (approved additive 620), Monopotassium L-glutamate (approved additive 622), and Calcium di-L-glutamate (approved additive 623).

Tartrazine (Approved Additive No 102)

This is a food dye used to colour foods yellow or orange. The scientific case against it is far less clear-cut than against metabisulphite, for instance. However, it can certainly do no harm to minimise exposure to foods coloured with it as much as possible. Such foods may include:

- Sweet syrups, toppings and savoury sauces
- Fruit juices
- Cordials
- Lollies
- Soft drinks
- Pickles
- Savoury snack foods
- Cakes, biscuits and baked goods
- Medicines coloured yellow, orange or green

Another dye which may also cause problems is Yellow 2G (approved additive 107).

SPOTTING THE BADDIES

This isn't always easy – not all foods listed above will necessarily contain the additives in question; while others, that are not listed, may contain them. Some foods contain more than one of the suspect additives. So how are you supposed to work out which to avoid?

A general rule of thumb is that fresh is best (though not always – the 'fresh' fruit salad you buy at food bars may have had its appearance enhanced with a dollop of metabisulphite). Remember that processed foods (canned, dried, frozen and precooked), takeaways and snack foods, all of which have to look good and last for a while on the shop shelf or counter, are likely to be high in these additives.

If your diet does include such processed foods (and there wouldn't be too many people whose doesn't), try to get into the habit of reading packet labels to work out <u>exactly</u> what's in them. Additives are often expressed in the form of numbers, as shown with those additives described above, so it makes sense to invest in a food additive code cracker. These are available from dieticians' offices, consumer organisations and the Department of Health, as well as from the National Asthma Campaign (for contacts, see page 85).

Chapter 4
Teamwork: Your Doctor and You

Denial – refusing to recognise the full implications of a disease – can be a big problem with asthma. This is understandable – who wants to worry about their health? – but can have tragic consequences if asthma is not controlled and treated properly. Much of the information in this book is particularly relevant to people with moderate or severe asthma, but it must be stressed that *all* asthmatics should have their condition assessed and treated on a regular basis by a doctor.

The majority of asthma cases are relatively mild. It is, however, a **chronic** disease, which means that you're likely to be stuck with it for a long period of time. And it is incurable, in the sense that your airways remain hypersensitive, even though you may not be suffering from acute attacks at a given point in time.

Because it can be such an insidious illness – asthmatics may feel quite well, without realising how much their lung function has been impaired – asthma should never be underestimated. A dangerous, possibly even fatal, attack is more likely to strike if the asthmatic has been turning a blind eye to his or her condition.

That's why it's essential that you develop a good relationship with your doctor and tackle your asthma together as a team. Because asthma is a disease requiring long-term monitoring, you should try to visit the same doctor as much as possible, so that he or she can build up a full picture of how you are dealing with it.

DIAGNOSIS

If you or your child are experiencing a respiratory problem, the first port of call should be a visit to your GP for diagnosis. Because asthma symptoms can be fairly dramatic – loud wheezing, breathlessness – you may have a good idea of what the problem is before you reach the doctor's surgery (though this is not necessarily the case, as we've seen; coughing, particularly at night, may be the *only* symptom of asthma, and this is a symptom that many people tend to downplay or ignore).

WHAT YOUR DOCTOR MAY DO

As it's likely that you won't be experiencing symptoms at the time you're seeing the doctor –

given that attacks are most common at night or early in the morning – he or she will probably ask you to describe them. He or she will also ask you when they occur, and whether they come on or worsen with exercise.

The doctor will probably also be interested in certain other aspects of your experience, such as:

- **History:** You may be asked about any family history of asthma, because of its hereditary component, and of other allergic complaints, such as hay fever and eczema, either in yourself or relatives.
- **Your lung function:** The doctor will examine you and will probably measure your lung function to see if it is impaired. This may be done with a **peak flow meter**, a hand-held device with a gauge on the side into which you blow (more about peak flow meters in Chapter 6). The gauge gives a numerical value to the rate at which you exhale; this is called your **peak expiratory flow** (PEF). This gives the doctor an idea of whether asthma is present (or how severe it is), by seeing how difficult you find it to breathe out. The greater the narrowing of the bronchi and the bigger the build-up of mucus, the harder it is to exhale. This test will probably be repeated a number of times to get the fullest picture of how the lungs are coping.
- **Your response to asthma medication:** If your PEF indicates that you have a problem, the

doctor may administer a **bronchodilator** (medication which opens up the airways), and then measure your lung function again. If it has now improved, it is likely that you have asthma.

The doctor may organise other tests, such as:

- **Your reaction to exercise:** Because asthma attacks can be triggered by exercise (see Chapter 8), your lung function may be measured before and after physical activity, to see if it deteriorates. If it does, this is another indicator that you have asthma. This test should be performed in a hospital or laboratory, where any resulting asthma attack can be promptly and properly treated.
- **Your reaction to allergens:** You may be asked to inhale substances which commonly trigger asthma attacks – such as dust or pollen – and your reaction observed. This is called an **asthma provocation test**, and, again, should be performed in a hospital or laboratory, to cope with any resulting asthma attack.
- **Chest X-ray:** If the bronchi have become blocked with mucus, air can be trapped within parts of the lungs. Other parts of the lungs may have deflated or collapsed because air can no longer reach them past the blockage. Both air trapping and lung collapse will show up on the X-ray, and are signs of asthma. Given the desirability

of keeping the body's exposure to X-rays to a minimum, however, a chest X-ray should not be the first or most likely method of diagnosis.

ASTHMA ASSESSMENT

Asthma varies in intensity quite considerably. Some people are relatively untroubled by it, others suffer frequent, disabling attacks. Your doctor will assess the severity of your asthma based on the information he or she has gained from physical examination, tests, your medical history and general day-to-day symptoms.

Asthma is graded as follows:

- **Mild:** Lung function normal most of the time; occasional symptoms, during exercise, for instance, or after infections; easily controlled by intermittent use of bronchodilators.
- **Moderate:** The asthmatic experiences regular and frequent symptoms; coughs at night; requires preventative medication, such as Intal or inhaled corticosteroids to control condition, but functions normally as long as daily medication is taken. More on medication in the next chapter.
- **Severe:** Wheezing and breathlessness with normal activities; the asthmatic is woken at night by wheezing, choking or breathlessness; requires high dose anti-inflammatory

medication, such as oral steroids; has required hospitalisation several times over the last five years.

- **Life-threatening:** The asthmatic wakes at night needing medication; has lost consciousness during attacks; has required ventilation (artificial breathing); does not respond well to bronchodilators. Out of control asthma is sometimes called **status asthmaticus**.

THE AIM OF TREATMENT

Whatever the grade of asthma, the treatment objective is the same:

- To keep lung function as close as possible to normal.
- To reduce asthma symptoms.
- To reduce the incidence and severity of attacks.

This objective may be achieved by a combination of:

- Medication (see Chapter 5).
- Monitoring lung function (see Chapter 6).
- Avoiding known asthma triggers as much as practicable, as detailed in Chapters 2 and 3.

ASTHMA MANAGEMENT PLAN

The National Asthma Campaign recommends this six-point Asthma Management Plan to doctors treating asthmatics:

1. **Assess severity of asthma.** This is done when the patient is well, not during an attack.

2. **Achieve best lung function.** Lung function is measured with a peak flow meter or spirometer. The doctor will then administer anti-asthma medication to get your lungs to function as well as possible. This is your best lung function, and the aim of treatment is to keep your normal lung function as close to that as possible.

3. **Avoid trigger factors.**

4. **Maintain lung function with optimal medication.** Your doctor will prescribe the lowest dosage and least medication necessary to maintain your lung function to your best level.

5. **Develop an action plan.** A written guide detailing appropriate reaction to asthma attacks.

6. **Education and regular review.** This means making sure that you and your family understand the objectives and methods of asthma control, and liaise at regular intervals with the doctor or medical support team.

TEAMWORK IS ESSENTIAL

As we've seen, many asthmatics who feel quite well actually have narrowing of the airways.

They may not be aware of the need for regular treatment, and never go near their doctor. It's important to take medication regularly, not just during an acute attack, to keep the airways open. This is why it's vital to see your doctor regularly for check-ups, not just during acute attacks. He or she should provide you with written crisis management instructions – concise information on what to do if the asthma suddenly worsens.

On the following pages you will find a suggested **asthma action plan** which you can take along to your doctor so that your individual needs can be written down.

Studies of asthma fatalities indicate that those who died tended not to have had a regular doctor advising them and monitoring their condition, and tended to underestimate and self-medicate their condition. But you and your doctor must co-operate if your asthma is to be successfully managed.

Your Asthma Action PLan

• What medication to take	
• How often it should be taken	
• When you should increase the dose	
• When to get medical help	
• What symptoms warrant all of the above	
• Emergency contact numbers	

It's easy to panic during an asthma attack – whether it's happening to yourself or a relative – and panicky people aren't normally noted for quick thinking. You can increase your chances of reacting promptly and appropriately if you have a written action plan handy. This plan

Fill in Together with Your Doctor

should be devised by your doctor specifically for you. It is designed to allow you to recognise when your asthma is getting worse and what action is then required. It should in effect talk you through the various stages of an attack.

Chapter 5
All About Medication

Now that your asthma has been diagnosed and assessed, what's next? As we've seen, the aim of treatment is to reduce attacks and keep lung function as close to normal as possible. This is achieved with a combination of careful monitoring, certain self-help measures, and, most importantly, medication.

Depending on the severity of your asthma, the doctor may prescribe:

1. Medications which will relieve asthma symptoms and arrest attacks.
2. Medications which treat asthma over the long term but will not stop attacks.

Some asthmatics will be able to get by with the first type alone; others will need both types of medication.

DRUGS THAT RELIEVE ASTHMA ATTACKS

Bronchodilators – medications which open up narrowed airways and make breathing easier –

are used to control asthma symptoms and ease wheezing during attacks. These are very effective and generally safe drugs. Asthmatics are advised to carry bronchodilator inhalers with them at all times, particularly while exercising, to help them cope with a sudden attack.

There are three main categories of bronchodilator:

- **Beta agonists:** These are sometimes referred to as 'sympathomimetics', meaning that they mimic the actions of adrenaline. Adrenaline is a hormone produced within the body which is responsible for the 'fight or flight' reaction: it opens up the airways to get more oxygen into the lungs to allow fast physical reactions at times of danger. Once, adrenaline itself was used to treat asthma; beta agonists are safer and better. They work by relaxing the muscles of the airways, and help clear mucus. Available as aerosols ('puffers' which deliver a metered dose, inhaled through the mouth), syrup, tablets, capsules which are inhaled and nebulising solution (see page 47 for explanation of methods of taking medication). *Brand names:* Berotec, Bricanyl, Ventolin, Salbuvent. *Possible side effects include:* Anxiety, tremors, increased heartbeat. **Note:** Use only one brand of beta agonist at a time. However, beta agonists can be taken with other types of bronchodilator, such as Theophylline or Atrovent (see below).

- **Theophylline:** This also works by relaxing the smooth muscles of the airways, making breathing easier. It is usually used with beta agonists, not alone. Available in tablets and syrups, and as slow-release tablets. *Brand names:* Choledyl, Nuelin, Biophylline, Labophylline, Lasma, Slo-phyllin, Pro-vent, Theo-Dur. *Possible side effects include:* Nausea and gastric upsets, palpitations and anxiety, headaches and loss of balance.

CAUTION

Many asthmatics become over-reliant on their bronchodilators, neglecting other, more appropriate, treatment. Because bronchodilator puffers can afford such quick relief, asthmatics may fail to monitor their lung function and be unaware that their condition may be deteriorating. It helps to keep an asthma diary (see Chapter 6) to keep track of just **how much** you are taking, and **how often**. You should consult your doctor if you find you are needing to use your puffer more often, or if each dose doesn't last for at least three or four hours. If so, you need to review your treatment. This is particularly so if you find asthma symptoms, such as coughing at night, are **increasing** or that your lung function is **deteriorating** (more on monitoring lung function in the following chapter). In such cases, **consult your doctor**.

- **Atrovent:** Also works by relaxing the muscles of the airways and preventing bronchial spasm. It also is usually used together with beta agonists, not alone. Available as an aerosol and nebulising solution. *Brand name:* Atrovent (this is the only drug in its class). *Possible side effects (rare) include:* Dry mouth, urinary retention.

DRUGS THAT TREAT ASTHMA BY PREVENTING ATTACKS RATHER THAN RELIEVING ATTACKS

There are other medications which are used on a long-term basis as a general preventative measure to make the airways less sensitive and reduce the risk of future attacks. Unlike bronchodilators, these drugs can't relieve the symptoms of an attack in progress.

Such medications fall into two categories:

- **Sodium cromoglycate:** This reduces the sensitivity of the mast cells lining the airways, inhibiting the release of histamines. It may be used before exercise to prevent exercise-induced asthma. *Brand name:* Intal. Available as an aerosol, capsule to be inhaled, nebuliser solution. *Possible side effects:* Virtually none, though it may cause coughing on talking. This is an extremely useful and effective medication. However, it must be taken every day to work properly, and it works slowly. It may be some time before results show.

- **Inhaled Corticosteroids:** These are forms of cortisone taken by aerosol or by capsules for inhalation, which reduce inflammation, mucus production and swelling of the breathing passages. They are topical medication (meaning they are applied directly to the problem area). When inhaled, they coat the airways, reducing their hypersensitivity. Corticosteroids may be prescribed if Intal is not effective, and are used to treat more severe asthma. Again, they have to be taken for some time before results may be noticeable. *Brand names:* Becotide, Pulmicort, Becloforte, Aldecin. *Possible side effects include:* thrush, sore throat, voice changes (these may be minimised by rinsing your mouth after taking – be sure not to swallow the rinse water – and by using a large volume spacer. See 'How Medication is Taken'.

  Some people with severe asthma may need to take cortisone tablets (oral steroids), usually for short periods of time. It is better not to take them over a long period, as used to be done before recent advances in asthma medication, because of possible serious side effects. The new strengthened dosage delivered by inhaled corticosteroids, such as Becloforte, may reduce or eliminate the need for oral steroid medication. *Brand names:* Prednisone, Prednisolone. *Possible side effects include:* (with prolonged use) Bloating, abnormal hair growth, retarded growth, osteoporosis, bruising, eye problems. *Note:*

Such side effects are unlikely since these medications are given in short courses, usually to reduce inflammation during and after asthma attacks, in which case their benefits outweigh the relatively slight risks.

CAUTION

Asthma medication should be taken as prescribed. DO NOT discontinue taking it because you feel well. Preventative treatment may have to be taken continuously to maintain lung function and protect you from future serious attacks. If you are unhappy with your medication, discuss it with your doctor. He or she may wish to review it from time to time.

Never go anywhere without your bronchodilator puffer — this is vitally important in case of a sudden asthmatic attack.

HOW MEDICATION IS TAKEN

Not only is there a seemingly bewilderingly large number of asthma medications, there are also several ways in which they can be taken. The primary aim of most asthma medication is to get it directly into the lungs, so it can quickly get to work where it is most needed. This is not always appropriate or possible, however. Medication may be taken by:

- **Aerosols:** These are an excellent way of treating asthma because they deliver medication right to the lungs, where they will do the most good. However, they require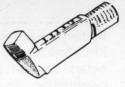

Aerosol

fairly good co-ordination, as the puffer must be 'pumped' and the spray inhaled simultaneously (ask your doctor to check your technique, to see that you're using your puffer properly). This makes puffers physically difficult to use for some people, such as the very young, the very old and the disabled.

- **Spinhaler, Rotahaler, Turbuhaler:** These are devices into which you insert a capsule of powdered medication at one end. The device splits the capsule and the powder is then inhaled through the other end. They are easier to use than **Turbuhaler** puffers, but still require a more precise inhalation technique than spacers (see below).

- **Spacers:** These are plastic devices into which metered-dose aerosols are inserted, with a chamber which retains the spray for you to inhale. Simultaneous co-ordination is not required; you pump the aerosol, then breathe in. Spacers may have small or large chambers.

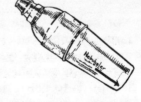

A Large Volume Spacer

FACT FILE

Puffers under Fire

Bronchodilator aerosols are popular with asthmatics because they relieve symptoms of breathlessness fast. But they have come under fire from some asthma experts, who believe they may worsen the asthma attack because

they open the airways to whatever is irritating them and causing the attack in the first place. It is thought that puffers may even contribute to asthma deaths: the use of such drugs has increased by 30 per cent since 1983 — a period in which asthma deaths have risen sharply in many industrialised countries. The high mortality figures could be coincidental (the worse an individual's asthma, the more likely he is to use a puffer, after all). Anyone who regularly relies on such puffers — particularly anyone using them daily — needs other treatment to control his or her asthma.

Beta agonists should be used under medical supervision.

- **Nebuliser:** A face mask through which an electric motor pumps a fine mist, to be inhaled, from a reservoir of liquid medication. It requires no particular co-ordination skills to use, and nebulisers may be purchased for use in the home. They are particularly useful during severe asthma attacks. **Important note:** Home nebulisers have come

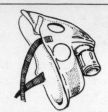

Nebuliser face mask

under attack from some respiratory experts, who believe that asthmatics experiencing severe attacks rely on using them when they should be heading for hospital. This can mean that their condition may deteriorate alarmingly before they call an ambulance.

- **Tablets and syrups:** Particularly used for medicating very small children.

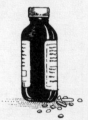

Tablets and syrups

Chapter 6
Monitoring Your Lung Function

The greatest single advance in the treatment of asthma in recent years is the wide availability of peak flow meters (sometimes referred to as PEF meters – short for Peak Expiratory Flow). These are available on prescription, and allow asthmatics to monitor their own lung function at home. They are basically hand-held tubes, with a gauge on the side, into which you blow. They are extremely easy to use.

Your doctor may use a peak flow meter to measure your lung capacity during consultations (and probably used one to help diagnose your asthma in the first place).

However, he or she doesn't often see you at the height of an attack (typically at night or early in the morning), so self-measurement with a peak flow meter lets him know exactly how severe the attack was. It also lets you know how you are doing – and how well you are managing your asthma.

HOW DO PEAK FLOW METERS WORK?

It is the effort of breathing out through narrowed airways that produces the characteristic asthmatic wheeze, as we've seen.

A peak flow meter is designed to check on the degree of difficulty experienced during exhaling. It does this by measuring how much air you can blow out after taking a deep breath. This is called your peak expiratory flow. The gauge gives a numerical reading for each exhalation. This measurement will vary depending on whether you are breathing easily or in the middle of an attack, and even on the time of day. Your job is to measure how often and when your lung capacity falls below that considered normal for your age, height and sex. You will know what this is from charts provided with the PEF monitor at purchase. (They are also available from chemists or through your doctor or the National Asthma Campaign – see page 86.)

Peak flow meter

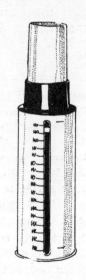

Your Personal Best

Monitoring your own lung capacity doesn't just allow you to compare your lung-function with that of other, non-asthmatic people. It also lets you see how your lungs are functioning compared with your own personal best PEF reading. Your doctor will help you establish what this is. If your PEF readings fall too far below that – lower than 50 per cent of your best after using a bronchodilator – you are in trouble and should get to your doctor or hospital fast.

How Often Should I Use My Peak Flow Meter?

Get into the habit of measuring your lung function twice a day – in the morning (when it's likely to be at its lowest) and again in the evening. On each occasion, blow into the peak flow meter three times, and make a note of the best reading thus obtained.

It helps to make a graph of your results and incorporate it into an asthma diary (see pages 55–6).

If the time you use your PEF meter coincides with the time you use your puffer, you should take a reading both before and shortly after (about 10–15 minutes) using the puffer. If you are taking medication in the form of tablets or syrup, wait up to an hour-and-a-half before taking another reading.

You should also use your peak flow meter during exercise to assess the impact physical activity is having on your lung function (more on exercise in Chapter 8).

Most importantly, you should use it during attacks, to see whether your lung function is deteriorating, a danger sign (see Chapter 7: 'Emergency – Coping with an Asthma Attack').

'I Feel Fine – Do I *Really* Need to Use a Peak Flow Meter?'

Many asthmatics feel great between attacks, but their lung function may have deteriorated quite considerably without their being aware of it. They need treatment to arrest this process and prevent the damage becoming permanent. The worse your lung capacity, the greater your risk of serious, and even potentially deadly, asthma attacks. Using a peak flow meter also allows you to monitor and assess how much your asthma reacts to medication. By revealing reduced lung capacity, it can give you advance warning of an impending attack. The more you know about your condition, the better you and your doctor will be able to manage it. Your peak flow meter is your best friend in this regard.

It is true that not everybody needs to use a peak flow meter regularly, depending on how mild and well controlled the asthma is. You should discuss your own case with your doctor and follow his or her recommendations. As a general rule of thumb, however, anybody whose asthma requires daily medication should be using a peak flow meter every day.

KEEPING A RECORD: YOUR 'ASTHMA DIARY'

Using your peak flow meter to monitor your lung function on a day-to-day basis is all very well, to gauge your reaction to treatment, exercise, and so on, but you should also use the information thus gathered to build up a picture of how your asthma is being controlled over the long term. The best way to do this is to keep an asthma diary – a daily record of all aspects of your asthma management. It should include such details as:

- Peak flow meter readings.
- How much medication was taken, and when.
- Asthma symptoms, such as coughing, wheezing, breathlessness.
- Whether you woke with symptoms, or they disturbed your sleep.
- Whether exercise brought on asthma symptoms.
- Time, place and circumstances of asthma attacks.

You should show this diary to your doctor. Such a record will help him or her identify factors precipitating attacks, as well as let him or her keep track of your response to medication.

Keeping an asthma diary is particularly useful for parents of asthmatic children. Young children often aren't able to give a very clear picture of their symptoms. When they're feeling fine, they may not even remember how they felt during an attack. More on children and asthma in Chapter 9.

MY ASTHMA DIARY

Keep a daily record like this for your and your doctor's information.

DATE _____

PEF meter reading (morning) _____

PEF meter reading (evening) _____

Medication taken _____

How much taken _____

When taken _____

ASTHMA SYMPTOMS:

Coughing	Yes/No
Wheezing	Yes/No
Breathlessness	Yes/No
Sleep disturbance	Yes/No
Did you wake with symptoms?	Yes/No

EXERCISE:

Did exercise bring on symptoms?	Yes/No

Type of exercise _____
_____

ASTHMA ATTACKS:

When did attack occur? _____

Where? _____

Give details _____
_____
_____
_____

Chapter 7
Emergency: Coping with an Asthma Attack

Asthma attacks often occur at night. They may take several hours to develop, or they may seem to blow up in a flash. They can vary in intensity quite considerably. Some are so mild they pass quickly without your having to do anything more than sit quietly for a minute or two. Others are so severe the person requires hospitalisation, and can even die. This is why it's important to have a written action plan that tells you how to respond properly to different levels of attack. Treat each one seriously, and don't be tempted to underestimate an attack, however mild it may turn out to be. You should be particularly on the alert for signs that your condition is deteriorating (by checking your peak flow meter).

Signs of an acute attack include:

- Coughing.
- Noisy wheezing.
- Tight chest.

- Breathlessness, even while resting.
- Sweating and shakiness.
- A choking feeling which fails to respond to bronchodilators.
- Your peak flow meter is showing the lowest level set by your doctor (see Chapter 6: 'Monitoring Your Lung Function').
- Labouring muscles under the rib cage.
- Feelings of anxiety, distress, sometimes confusion.

The most important thing is to remain calm – if you panic, this may only intensify the severity of the attack. Sit upright; this will make it easier for you to breathe. Don't forget to use your peak flow meter to help you gauge the severity of the attack.

Medication is your first line of defence against an asthma attack. Because your airways are narrowed and even blocked, making it difficult for medication to get through, the usual tactic is to *increase* your normal dose of bronchodilator – preferably by nebuliser, because this delivers a bigger dosage than an aerosol. Bronchodilators may be taken every three or four hours during attacks. Because extra inflammation is a characteristic of an acute asthma attack, oral steroids such as Prednisolone (*not* aerosol steroids) may be taken, according to your doctor's instructions. It will take some time for you to feel the effect, but they may ultimately shorten the attack.

If, however, you're still in distress 15 minutes

after first using your bronchodilator, try again. If there's still no response within another 10 minutes or so, call your GP immediately, or call an ambulance. Don't attempt to drive to hospital – this is a medical emergency, and it is better to call an ambulance. Remember to specify that you are suffering an asthma attack when calling the ambulance.

Important: These are general observations concerning medication for acute asthma attack, and are not a substitute for your own asthma action plan and your own doctor's advice.

WHAT HAPPENS NEXT

You are likely to be given Ventolin and Atrovent by nebuliser at hospital or in your GP's surgery. If you're still not responding, you may be given a steroid injection to reduce inflammation, particularly if you're showing signs of **cyanosis** – that is, your nose, lips and fingers are turning blue from lack of oxygen. In hospital you may also be given a **blood gas test** to determine the relative concentrations of oxygen and carbon dioxide in your blood. This test shows how advanced the asthma is, because, over time, asthmatics become able to tolerate lower levels of oxygen and higher levels of carbon dioxide than normal.

WHEN TO GET MEDICAL HELP

Nobody likes making a fuss, particularly if it turns out to be unwarranted. And nobody's very keen on going to hospital. Some asthmatics may hang back from getting medical assistance at the appropriate time for either of these reasons, or because they don't recognise the potential seriousness of their symptoms. So how do you know when to hit the panic button?

You should *always* seek medical attention if:

- You're not responding to bronchodilators or the doses you've taken don't last at least two hours.
- You've had severe asthma attacks or been hospitalised before (this makes you a higher risk patient).
- The attack started very suddenly (more common in uncontrolled asthma).
- You're *very* breathless.
- You're worried in any way.
- You notice signs of cyanosis (blueness, as above).

Remember that wheezing is not invariably a sign of an acute asthma attack. In some cases of severe asthma it may not be particularly noticeable, but you may still be in considerable distress.

Don't be shy about summoning assistance, even if you feel you could be overreacting.

Many asthma deaths occur in people who have dangerously underestimated the severity of their condition, and medical personnel would far rather be confronted with someone who has panicked unnecessarily than someone beyond their help.

Chapter 8
Exercise for Asthmatics

Exercise, as we've seen in Chapter 2, can trigger asthma attacks (this is called **exercise induced asthma**, or **EIA**). In fact, wheezing after physical activity is one of the key symptoms of asthma, which is why your doctor is likely to ask about your reaction to exercise when diagnosing your condition. EIA is particularly common in children, because they are active by nature and tend to run around more than adults.

WHAT CAUSES EIA?

Most forms of exercise make you breathe more heavily and quickly. This means, among other things, that larger quantities than usual of cold, dry air are passing over the airways, drying out the mucus membranes and irritating them – which can trigger an asthma attack.

The risks of EIA are increased by exercising:

- In cold, dry air.
- During at-risk times, such as during the pollen season.

- When you have a cold or other respiratory infection.

SHOULD ASTHMATICS REFRAIN FROM EXERCISE?

Those whose asthma is unstable (not responding to medication, for instance, or waking them at night) may have to avoid exercise, according to their doctor's advice. But in general, those whose asthma is well controlled will be encouraged to undertake physical activity. This is because exercise has a great many health benefits, including increasing lung capacity and cardiac fitness, and reducing stress. Some exercises, such as swimming, are particularly good for asthmatics.

Exercise has important psychological benefits, too. Asthmatics, particularly children, should not be encouraged to consider themselves invalids or to impose limitations upon their potential achievements (this doesn't mean asthmatics should ignore or downplay their condition – just keep it in perspective).

Regular, healthy exercise can also impart a great sense of achievement and well-being.

In any case, the risk of EIA can be reduced by taking medication *before* commencing physical activity (more about this below).

WHICH EXERCISE IS RIGHT FOR ME?

This is an individual decision – only **you** know, for certain, how you react to various activities. In general, you should do exercise that you enjoy and are likely to keep up. If you like walking, walk. If tennis or golf is your game, give it a go.

That being said, you should be aware that certain types of exercise are more likely to trigger attacks than others. Skiing is particularly hazardous, because it typically involves strenuous exercise performed over long periods in cold air. And prolonged running, particularly in cool air, is more likely to provoke an attack than 'stop-start' activities, such as tennis doubles.

It goes without saying that you should **consult your doctor** before starting any exercise regime.

Don't just plunge willy-nilly into an ambitious activity programme – this could be dangerous if you are prone to EIA. Your doctor can advise you on the amount and type of exercise that is appropriate for your condition and level of fitness.

EXERCISE TO AVOID

Asthmatics should not do any exercise in which they can't use medication, if and when required. For instance, a sport like scuba diving is definitely out, and as we've seen above, you should be cautious about exercising in cold, dry air.

HOW TO EXERCISE

1. Make It Regular
While exercise can trigger attacks, they may

decrease with regular exercise. The more you exercise, the fitter you become and the less oxygen you will need to perform the same amount of physical activity.

In other words, you won't need to breathe as heavily as when you were less fit – which means that less cold air is flowing over your airways and irritating them. Result: fewer asthma attacks. You are still susceptible to EIA, but at a more intense level of exercise – so ordinary exercise shouldn't affect you as much.

So how much exercise do you need? The more the better, but, as a rule of thumb, you should try to exercise at least three times a week for at least 30 minutes at a time.

FACT FILE

Did You Know?
Asthma hasn't stopped several athletes reaching the top of their profession, even Olympian standard. For instance, champion marathon swimmer Susie Maroney, who successfully completed a double crossing of the English Channel in 1990, was advised to take up swimming to help her childhood asthma.

2. Make a Splash

Swimming has special benefits for asthmatics because it teaches breath control. It also takes place in a moist environment – obviously! –

which doesn't dry out the mucus membranes as much as some other exercises.

And you're hardly likely to be kicking up allergens like dust and pollen, as you may in other sports played on grass, such as cricket or football. Swimming in a heated pool seems to be particularly beneficial. Contact the National Asthma Campaign for information on swimming classes for asthmatics (see page 86).

3. Prevention of EIA

The more open the airways, the less likely EIA is to develop. So attacks may be warded off by taking medication immediately before commencing exercise: several puffs of Ventolin or Intal, according to your doctor's directions, a few minutes before the game or activity in question.

Note: This is in addition to your normal dosage. People using such medication daily or several times a day could organise their exercise schedule to coincide with the time they would normally be taking their medication. That way, you don't have to increase your total daily intake.

4. Warming Up First

The risk of EIA may also be decreased if activity is preceded by a short warm-up period in the half hour or so before the proper exercise is commenced.

A 'cooling down' period afterwards also

seems to be helpful. The aim is not to plunge suddenly into vigorous activity and then stop again just as suddenly, but to build up to an exercise level, then slowly wind down.

5. Keep Your Nose Clear

Asthmatics should try to breathe through their noses whenever possible, because the nose filters, warms and humidifies air before it arrives at the lungs. The mouth is not as efficient an 'air-conditioner' as the nose, and mouth-breathing results in colder, drier air being delivered to the lungs, irritating the airways. While it's virtually impossible not to pant through open mouth during heavy exercise, you should try to avoid this as much as possible during lighter activities, such as walking. If exercise tends to block your nose – a common situation – you could unblock it with a nasal decongestant. If you're not too keen on becoming a walking chemist's shop every time you want to work out – carrying decongestants and puffers – you could try wearing a surgical-style mask during exercise. This can help prevent your nose becoming blocked in the first place (though it may make you look like the Lone Ranger!)

MEASURING YOUR PERFORMANCE

As well as sprays, it could be a good idea sometimes to carry your peak flow meter when exercising, so that you can measure lung function before, during and after exercise, to see how it is responding to the activity (and medication).

If, during exercise, you find that your flow rate has dropped below 75 per cent of normal or resting rate, you should discuss the situation with your doctor.

This being said, it's worth pointing out that it is not necessarily practicable nor even desirable always to carry a peak flow meter during sport – it may make children feel 'different' and self-conscious, for example – so ask your doctor whether it's warranted in your case.

Stop/start activities such as tennis are less likely to trigger exercise-induced asthma than other, sustained activities such as running or skiing.

Chapter 9
Children and Asthma

Asthma is very much a childhood disease, afflicting about one in seven British children to some degree at some time during their childhood. It is the most common childhood lung disease.

Why are young children so prone to asthma? Their airways are smaller than adults', which makes them more easily obstructed or blocked by airway narrowing and mucus. And children's immune systems are less developed than adults', making them more susceptible to environmental irritants. This is one reason for an important difference between childhood asthma and adult asthma. Childhood asthma is much more clearly an **atopic** (allergic) disease; nearly twice as many asthmatic children as asthmatic adults are generally 'allergic'.

Another factor is young children's greater susceptibility to infection. Colds and other respiratory ailments are very common in children under the age of five, and such infections commonly trigger asthma attacks. However, a child becomes less susceptible to infections as he or she grows older, and so the number of asthma attacks should decline over time.

CHILDREN AT RISK

Pre-school children have the highest incidence of asthma; it drops away steeply after the age of 10, as children become immune to the majority of respiratory viruses as they grow. Boys are affected by childhood asthma at twice the rate of girls; this ratio is reversed after puberty, with girls more susceptible.

However, attacks may stop altogether by puberty or young adulthood. Such children are said to have 'grown out of' their asthma, but their airways still have a tendency to hypersensitivity, and there is still some risk of asthma attacks. Some people can have an attack after 40 years free of them.

A small proportion of asthmatic children will continue to suffer asthma attacks into adulthood.

ASSESSING CHILDHOOD ASTHMA

Despite the alarming statistics, the overwhelming majority of asthmatic children – around 75 per cent – suffer **mild** or **episodic** asthma, controlled by intermittent use of bronchodilators (according to the doctor's advice). They don't need preventative medication between attacks. Lung function is usually normal between attacks, which only strike at intervals of several weeks or longer. (These attacks may still be quite severe, nevertheless, and may even require hospitalisation and additional medication.) Around half of these children appear to have grown away from their asthma by adolescence or adulthood.

A much smaller number – around 20 per cent of asthmatic children – have **moderate** asthma. Attacks are more frequent, and lung function often doesn't return to normal between attacks. They may need to take regular preventative medication between attacks.

A tiny percentage – under 5 per cent – suffer **severe** asthma. This means that they wheeze frequently, are woken by their asthma, have their activities limited and miss a lot of school because of it, respond poorly to bronchodilators, and require frequent hospitalisation. They need specialist care and regular medication (generally inhaled steroids and possibly oral steroids during attacks). Fortunately, such cases are in the minority.

The age at which asthma strikes seems to be relevant to the severity of asthma. If this is before the age of two, the asthma is likely to be more severe and to continue into adulthood.

FACT FILE

Problem Playthings
Fabric-covered 'cuddlies' and soft plush toys harbour dust. Plastic or wooden toys are better for asthmatic children (if less likely to be as 'loved'!)

CHILDREN AND ASTHMA MEDICATION

Small children usually take asthma medication by nebuliser or as syrup. Treatment is difficult for babies and toddlers, as the muscles of their airways are too immature to respond to bronchodilators, and they will probably need to be hospitalised during severe asthma attacks. They may take Intal inhaled through a nebuliser. They may also be given corticosteroids if considered necessary by their doctors.

Slightly older children respond to bronchodilator medication, but usually lack the co-ordination to use puffers properly. They may take bronchodilators by nebuliser or as syrup, and take Intal by nebuliser. Theophyllines may be given as a syrup.

By school age (or even younger), some children will be able to use volume spacers, rotahalers and other devices such as the Turbuhaler or Volumatic. Your doctor will be able to advise on when your child is capable of using an aerosol properly (usually around the age of 7 or so), and should teach him or her the proper technique.

MONITORING YOUR CHILD'S ASTHMA

As we've seen in Chapter 6, monitoring lung function with a PEF meter is the best and easiest way of keeping an eye on how asthma is being controlled. Very young children will need a modified version of a PEF meter. Obviously, if you notice that the child's peak rate is decreasing, it's time to seek further medical advice.

Other danger signs to watch out for:

- Increasing wheezing, chest tightness and coughing, particularly at night or first thing in the morning.
- The child needs to use his or her puffers more often.
- The child's physical activity is increasingly limited by asthma.
- The child is coming down with more respiratory infections, and/or seems generally miserable and off-colour.

All these indicate that the asthma is worsening, and it is time to review the child's management programme with the doctor.

COPING WITH YOUR CHILD'S ASTHMA ATTACKS

Try to keep as calm as possible, to help calm the child. In general, follow the guidelines outlined in Chapter 7, remembering to follow the child's own asthma action plan outlined by your doctor. Don't hesitate to get medical help if at all concerned.

AT SCHOOL

Starting school can be a worrying time for parents. It means several hours a day during which the child is out of your care, when you're not available to deal with any asthma attacks that may develop. It is essential that you discuss your child's condition and medication requirements fully with the head teacher and class teacher.

Whether or not your child will be allowed to carry his or her inhaler while at school is at the discretion of the head teacher. In some infant and primary schools the head teachers prefer that the inhalers are kept there by a responsible adult.

WHAT ABOUT PLAY TIME?

As we've seen, running around, particularly in cold air, can trigger asthma attacks, but that doesn't mean you should attempt to curtail your child's activity level. Boisterous physical activity is a normal part of childhood, and the child shouldn't be encouraged to see himself or herself as an invalid. It's better to get the child into the habit of using his or her bronchodilator puffer just before exercise – and possibly taking another puff during exercise, if required. Intal could be taken as well as, or instead of, a bronchodilator.

However, depending on the severity of the asthma, some children may have to refrain from physical activities sometimes. The child will learn to know his or her limitations, and should use his or her judgement. Teachers should be made aware that the child may have to be excused from sport and PE at times.

FACT FILE

Fat, Happy Wheezers

As every mother knows, babies are wheezy little things, due to the fact that their immature airways are still quite 'floppy'. Wheezing may be a key symptom of asthma, but 'all that wheezes is not (necessarily) asthma'. In general, if the baby looks well, puts on weight and doesn't seem upset by his wheezing, you probably have no cause for concern. Such babies are often called fat, happy wheezers, and the wheezing clears up as they grow older. However, you **should** seek medical advice if the baby's breathing is obviously laboured, if the wheezing is interfering with feeding and sleeping, and if asthma runs in the family.

PHYSICAL PROBLEMS

As long as a child's asthma is well controlled, he or she is unlikely to suffer permanent lung damage from attacks.

However, chronic, severe asthma from an early age may have certain physical repercussions. One is the 'barrel chest' or 'pigeon chest' deformity (enlarged chest and prominent breastbone) caused by lungs becoming permanently over-inflated due to difficulties in exhaling properly.

Another problem is growth retardation. This is sometimes blamed on use of steroidal medication, but seems to be a feature of many chronic childhood diseases, and is probably due to the illness, not the medication. The effects will not be permanent and the child will eventually catch up.

Improper breathing can lead to a hunched, round-shouldered posture; this can be improved by learning better breathing techniques.

EMOTIONAL ASPECTS

Taking medication, having to refrain from certain activities, and frequent absences from school all conspire to make the child feel different from his or her peers; and children who feel different can become self-conscious and withdrawn.

Anger, resentment, fear, depression and feelings of inferiority are all common reactions to chronic illness. These are tough emotions to cope with when you're still only a child.

It doesn't help that missing school can affect the child's academic progress; or that, when at school, he or she may be tired from disturbed nights; or that some asthma medications can cause anxiety, irritability and impaired concentration. Asthma can take a tremendous emotional toll on the whole family. The parents may focus their attention on the sick child, and siblings may feel resentful and left out. The whole household may seem to revolve around the child's asthma attacks, increasing his or her anxiety and feelings of difference.

These are very real problems and ones that are not easily dealt with. However, there is some evidence to suggest that the way the parents approach their child's asthma can affect the child's ability to cope. A calm, matter-of-fact approach to the illness tends to relieve the child's own fears.

Helping to build the child's self-esteem is important, as is gentle encouragement to participate in as many normal activities as possible. The National Asthma Campaign runs a junior asthma club which provides support specifically for children (see page 86).

'ONLY NERVY, NEUROTIC CHILDREN GET ASTHMA'

This is a myth, as we've seen, but one that all too many people still believe. Because stress does play a part in triggering attacks, it could be worth investigating events in the child's life, either at school or at home, which may be distressing him or her. It may also be a good idea to teach the child breathing and relaxing exercises, to help cope with the next attack. Your own anxiety level can be infectious; the child is far more likely to keep cool during an attack if you can.

INVOLVE THE CHILD

As with any chronic disease, it's a good idea to involve the child in the management of his or her asthma as much as possible. This means allowing him or her to monitor lung capacity when practicable, and entrusting him or her to take medication. It also means allowing the child to sit in on consultations with the doctor, and even to consult the doctor alone when old enough. This is part of the 'letting go' process, which all parents – even those with sick children – must undergo at some point.

THE TEENAGE YEARS

Adolescence can be a major headache for parents of asthmatics. Teenagers are struggling to establish their independence. They don't want to be seen as sick in any way, they don't want to have their physical activities curtailed, and they don't want to be bothered with aerosols and PEF meters and all the other asthma paraphernalia.

And they are preoccupied with self-image, which makes life very hard for that very small proportion of children with severe asthma whose physical development may have been delayed by their condition. This is a time of challenges to parental authority, and typical teenage rebellion may take the form of smoking – bad enough for anyone, but downright disastrous for asthmatics.

Non-compliance – failing to take medication or follow the asthma action plan – can become a real issue now. Parental nagging, while understandable, is likely to be counterproductive.

It doesn't help that adolescence can be a time

of emotional upheaval, and the resulting tension and anxiety may trigger or worsen asthma attacks in some individuals.

It is now that proper asthma education, started on diagnosis, can really pay off. The better the child understands his or her condition and the necessity for proper management from the word go, the more likely he or she is to comply.

A good relationship with a trusted doctor – one whom the teenager may consult alone – is helpful in this respect. This is why it is important that the child (and adult asthmatic, for that matter) continues to consult the same doctor, to allow a long-term picture of the individual's pattern of asthma to be built up. The more the doctor and asthmatic understand the condition, the more successfully it can be controlled – and the easier it is to live with asthma.

FACT FILE

Smoke Ring
The high incidence of asthma among today's children is often linked with increased industrial pollution. But a team of respiratory experts who carried out studies of a major city's smoggy suburbs declared pollution a long way down the list of asthma triggers. Parents who were heavy smokers were more likely culprits – producing their own form of air pollution within the home.

Glossary

It can sometimes seem as though doctors and asthma specialists speak a language of their own, full of words starting with 'broncho' and 'pulmonary'. Here are simple explanations of some terms asthmatics may encounter in the course of treatment.

Atopic: Allergic.

Allergens: Substances which trigger allergic reactions. Also called antigens.

Allergic rhinitis: Hay fever, an allergic condition with which asthma is associated.

Allergy: Hypersensitivity to certain substances (allergens), resulting from an overreaction of the immune system.

Alveoli: Tiny air sacs of the lungs.

Beta agonists: A type of bronchodilator medication (see below).

Bronchi: Major airways of the lungs which branch off from the windpipe.

Bronchioles: Smaller airways of the lungs which, in turn, branch off from the bronchi.

Bronchodilator: Medication which expands the

airways by relaxing their muscles; the first line of defence in an asthma attack.

Bronchospasm: Contraction of the smooth muscles of the airways, involved in asthma attacks.

Cilia: Tiny hairlike filaments lining the airways which move impurities up out of the lungs.

Cyanosis: When lack of oxygen causes lips, tongue, fingers and nose tip to turn blue; a sign that an asthma attack is dangerously severe and urgent medical attention is required.

Eczema: Inflammation of the skin, an allergic condition with which asthma is associated.

Histamines: Chemicals released from the body's mast cells on exposure to allergens.

Hyperventilation: Over-breathing, resulting in low carbon dioxide levels in the blood.

Lumen: The space in the centre of the airways, normally open to allow air through. With asthma, this space is narrowed and even blocked by muscle spasm and mucus production, making breathing difficult.

Mast cells: Special cells found throughout the body, particularly in the mucus membranes lining the airways, which release chemicals involved in allergic reactions.

Mucosa: A layer of special, mucus-producing cells lining the respiratory tract.

Nebuliser: Device which pumps liquid medication in a fine mist through a face mask for inhalation.

Pulmonary: To do with the lungs.

Pulmonary artery: Major blood vessel of the lung.

Pulmonary function test: Measuring lung capacity and function to determine the degree of asthma present. This is done with a machine called a spirometer, which measures how fast and how much air the person can exhale, or breathe out.

Pulmonary vein: Another important blood vessel of the lung.

RAST (Radioallergosorbent) test: A sophisticated allergy test which determines an individual's sensitivity to certain substances by measuring specific allergic antibodies in the blood.

Status asthmaticus: Uncontrolled asthma which does not respond to medication.

Thoracic: To do with the chest. For example, a thoracic surgeon is a chest specialist.

Trachea: Wind pipe.

Helpful Addresses

There are a number of organisations that give support and advice about the management of asthma in children and adults.

Action Against Allergy (AAA)
24/26 High Street
Hampton Hill
Middlesex
TW12 1PD
(Send a stamped addressed envelope for information)

Asthma Research Council
12 Penbridge Square
London
W2 4EH

British Lung Foundation
Kingsmead House
250 Kings Road
London
SW3 5UE
(0171) 371 7704

Chest, Heart and Stroke Association
55 North Castle Street
Edinburgh
EH2 3LT
(0131) 225 6963

General Practitioners in Asthma Group (GPIAG)
MM1
Bath Brewery
Toll Bridge Road
Bath
BA1 7DE
(01225) 858880

National Asthma Campaign
Providence House
Providence Place
London
N1 0NT
(01345) 010203 (Helpline)
(Runs a junior asthma club)

Pilgrims: The National School for Asthma/Eczema
Firle Street
Seaford
Sussex
BN25 2HX
(01323) 892697

Robinson Family Health

All your health questions answered in a way you really understand

Available from leading bookshops, or from Robinson using the order form below
or by writing to the address given

ORDER FORM

Please Tick

Arthritis: What Really Works
Dava Sobel & Arthur C Klein £7.99
"I cannot recommend this book too highly."
Dr James Le Fanu, Daily Telegraph

☐

Asthma: Breathe Easy
Megan Gressor £2.99

☐

Brain Damage: Don't Learn to Live With It!
Margaret Baker and Trevor England £7.99

☐

Bulima Nervosa & Binge Eating
Dr Peter Cooper £6.99
"Highly recommended." British Journal of Psychiatry

☐

The Good Diet Guide: Choose the diet that's right for you
Dr Jane Dunkeld £6.99

☐

Headaches: Relief at Last
Megan Gressor £2.99

☐

Massage for Common Ailments
Penny Rich £4.99 (full colour)

☐

Overcoming IBS
Dr Christine P Dancey and Susan Backhouse £6.99
"A simply excellent book" Dr James Le Fanu, Sunday Telegraph

☐

Practical Aromatherapy
Penny Rich £4.99 (full colour)

☐

The Recovery Book: A Life-saving Guide for Alcoholics and Addicts
Al J Mooney, A & H Eisenburg £9.99
"The most complete and accurate compendium I've ever read."
James W West, Betty Ford Centre

☐

Women's Waterworks: Curing Incontinence
Pauline Chiarelli £2.99

☐

You *Can* Beat Period Pain
Liz Kelly £2.99

☐

Orders to: Robinson Publishing Ltd., 7 Kensington Church Court, London W8 4SP

I enclose a cheque for £ _____ in payment for the books indicated above.
Post & Packing FREE within the UK, please add 20% for postage outside the UK.

Name: _____

Address: _____

_____ Postcode: _____

(Please allow 28 days for delivery in the UK, longer elsewhere)

☐ Tick here if you would like to receive information on new health titles from Robinson